EYE EXERCISE HANDBOOK

Beginners Guide To Vision Improvement & Enhancing Your Eye Health

VINCENT JERRY

Table of Contents

Introductory

The term "eye exercises" refers to a variety of techniques designed to improve visual acuity and eye health. Regularly performing these exercises will aid in reducing eye fatigue, improving eyesight, strengthening eye muscles, and enhancing overall eye health.

Eye exercises are designed to relax and strengthen the muscles responsible for eye movement, focus, and lens shape regulation. In addition, they can help increase oxygen to the eyes and reduce eye strain caused by activities such as prolonged reading or computer use.

Common eye exercises include:

• Excessive screen time can cause the eyes to become dry and irritated; therefore, it is necessary to exercise rapid or intentional blinking at regular intervals.

• Palming is a technique that involves rubbing your palms together to generate warmth and then placing them lightly over your closed eyelids to relax your eyes and relieve eye strain.

• Changing the focal distance from one object to another can help your eyes and muscles become more flexible and coordinated.

• Eye muscles can be exercised by rolling the eyeballs in various directions, including up and down, side to side, and in a circle.

• Concentrating on a nearby object and then a distant object is a wonderful way to strengthen the eyes' ability to focus and reduce eye strain.

However, eye exercises should not be viewed as a substitute for medical attention from a trained eye care professional; at best, they can provide temporary relief and assist in maintaining eye health.

If you have been experiencing persistent or severe vision problems, an optometrist or ophthalmologist can examine your eyes thoroughly and prescribe treatment.

CHAPTER ONE
Regarding The Eyes

Due to the significance of vision in our daily lives, maintaining excellent eye health is essential. Listed below are several reasons why it is essential to take care of your eyes:

• Good eyesight is necessary for experiencing the world around us, appreciating its splendor, and completely participating in the many available activities. Healthy eyesight significantly improves the capacity to read, drive, work, and engage in leisure activities.

- Routine eye examinations can detect eye disorders and diseases in their earliest stages, frequently before symptoms manifest. Because of this early detection and prompt treatment and care, the potential impact on a person's vision and overall eye health is lessened.

Untreated eye diseases and injuries, such as glaucoma, macular degeneration, and diabetic retinopathy, can result in irreversible vision loss. Vision loss can be prevented with meticulous attention to eye care and prompt treatment of problems.

• As a consequence of spending so much time staring at electronic devices, many people suffer from eye strain and pain. Taking care of our eyes while using a computer by taking frequent breaks, maintaining the proper distance from the screen, and utilizing proper illumination can significantly reduce eye strain and pain.

• A person's eye health may be indicative of their overall health and well-being. Eye changes are a prevalent sign of systemic diseases, such as diabetes and hypertension. In addition, a number of eye conditions can serve as indicators of broader health concerns. By caring for our eyes, we can detect issues early on and enhance our overall health.

• As we age, age-related ocular diseases are more likely to manifest. With early detection and treatment of age-related eye diseases such as cataracts, presbyopia, and age-related macular degeneration, improved vision and quality of life can be achieved in old age.

Maintaining one's safety and independence requires clear, healthy vision. As a consequence, we are better able to navigate, identify potential threats, and go about our daily lives without fear. Maintaining our independence and sense of safety is as simple as maintaining healthy eyes.

For maintaining good eye health, it is recommended to engage in appropriate eye care practices, such as wearing corrective lenses as prescribed, in addition to undergoing regular comprehensive eye examinations, living a healthy lifestyle (including a balanced diet, regular exercise, and proper eye protection), and managing chronic health conditions.

The Consequences Of Frequent Eye Problems

There are numerous common eye disorders, each with unique impacts on a person's eyesight and overall eye health. The most prevalent ocular conditions and their effects are as follows:

- Myopia (nearsightedness), hyperopia (farsightedness), astigmatism, and presbyopia are all refractive defects that impair the eye's ability to accurately focus light on the retina.

- These issues can result in hazy vision, difficulty focusing on adjacent or distant objects, and eye fatigue.

• Cataracts develop when the normal lens of the eye becomes opaque or cloudy. They can make it difficult to see in the dark, diminish colors, increase glare sensitivity, and more. Cataracts tend to develop progressively with age, but the cloudy lens can be replaced surgically.

• Increased intraocular pressure is a common symptom of glaucoma, a group of eye disorders characterized by injury to the optic nerve. It can cause permanent vision loss or even blindness in the affected eye(s) if left untreated.

• The primary target of age-related macular degeneration (AMD) is the degeneration of the macula, the portion of the retina most responsible for central vision. It can lead to a loss of central vision, making it difficult to read, identify features, and perform other tasks requiring sharp focus.

• Diabetic retinopathy, damage to the retinal blood vessels, is a serious complication of diabetes. In its advanced stages, age-related macular degeneration can cause complete and permanent vision loss due to blurred or wavy vision, black patches or floaters, difficulty distinguishing colors, and other symptoms.

• Dry eye syndrome can develop when the eyes do not produce sufficient tears or when the tears evaporate too rapidly. Possible adverse effects include dryness, itchiness, redness, a grainy sensation, and blurred vision. In extreme instances, corneal damage may result from untreated dry eye.

• The condition known colloquially as "pink eye" is caused by inflammation of the conjunctiva, the thin tissue that borders the inside of the eyelids and covers the whites of the eyes. Symptoms include blurred vision, itching, and discharge.

There are numerous potential causes of infectious conjunctivitis, including bacteria, viruses, allergens, and irritants.

These are only a few of the numerous symptoms and causes of prevalent eye diseases. Despite the fact that the severity of each condition differs from individual to individual, it is evident that early diagnosis and treatment are essential for preventing irreversible vision loss.

Regular eye exams with an optometrist or ophthalmologist can help detect these issues early so that they can be effectively addressed, resulting in improved eye health.

CHAPTER TWO
The Importance Of Eye Exercise

There are a number of potential advantages to eye exercises for eye health. Even though there is limited data on the benefits of eye exercises, many individuals have found that incorporating them into their routine has been beneficial. Among the potential benefits of eye exercises are the following:

• Regular eye exercises can reduce the strain on your eyes caused by gazing at a computer screen, a book, or any other visual stimulus for extended periods of time. They can alleviate eye strain and make you feel less fatigued and strained.

• Eye exercises that require alternating between close and far objects or following a moving target can improve concentration and focus.

• Like any other muscle in the body, eye muscles can be strengthened through exercise. Eye exercises are designed to improve the coordination and efficiency of the muscles responsible for concentration and eye movement.

• Eye muscle flexibility can be increased through exercises

requiring eye movement in various directions, such as rolling or tracing patterns.

• Despite the fact that eye exercises cannot directly improve visual acuity or correct refractive errors, some claim to have experienced temporary improvements in vision clarity and sharpness after engaging in specific eye exercises. These exercises may improve the way your brain processes visual information.

• By increasing blood flow to the eyes, eye exercises contribute to improved overall eye health by nourishing and oxygenating the eye tissues.

• In addition, specific eye exercises, such as blinking or palming, can alleviate dehydration and irritation of the eyes.

• The stress-relieving and mood-enhancing effects of deep breathing and palming, two common components of many eye exercises, are well-documented. Possibile benefits of these exercises include reduced stress and eye tension.

It is important to note that not everyone finds eye exercises beneficial or suitable for their requirements. Before commencing a new fitness program, if you have any preexisting eye diseases or conditions, you should consult an eye doctor.

Maintaining regular eye exams, proper eye care routines, and professional guidance for persistent or severe eye issues are also essential for ensuring good overall eye health.

Preparing For Eye Training

As part of preparing for eye exercises, you must ensure that you have a tranquil and comfortable space in which to practice. Consider the following points prior to commencing eye exercises:

• Choose a Calm Environment: It is essential to perform your eye exercises in an environment that is free of commotion and distractions. Keep distractions to a minimum and have adequate lighting available to prevent eye fatigue.

• Choose a time of day when you won't be interrupted and can devote your full attention to eye exercises. Try not to rush through them or perform too many tasks simultaneously.

• Prior to commencing your eye exercises, you may wish to engage in some mental and physical relaxation techniques. Try deep breathing exercises or progressive muscle relaxation to get into the zone for your workout.

• As with any other form of exercise, eye exercises can be made more effective by first warming up the involved muscles. Warm your hands by massaging them together, then rest them for a few minutes on your closed eyes. This benefits both the circulation to the eyes and the muscles surrounding them.

• Ensure that you are seated upright by adjusting your chair as necessary. Indirectly influencing eye health and comfort, poor posture can cause neck, shoulder, and back pain and discomfort.

• To maximize the effectiveness of your eye exercises, you should remove your spectacles or contact lenses. You can determine whether or not to wear your glasses based on the exercises you are performing and how you feel.

• Follow the prescribed techniques and movements for each eye exercise. Always read and strictly adhere to the exercise instructions. Each exercise's duration, cadence, and range of motion are crucial, so pay close attention to these factors.

• If you're going to perform a series of eye exercises, it's essential to give your eyes a 15- to 20-minute break between exercises. During these times, you can rest your eyes by closing them, gazing into the distance, or performing other gentle eye relaxation techniques.

Remember that you should only perform as many eye exercises as is comfortable. Stop performing the exercises and consult an eye doctor if you experience pain or discomfort.

Even if you regularly perform eye exercises, it is essential to visit an optometrist or ophthalmologist for regular examinations in order to maintain good eye health. These specialists will provide you with specific suggestions for enhancing your eye health.

Creating A Pleasing Visual Environment

Maintaining healthy eyes and reducing eye strain necessitate a pleasurable environment for the eyes. Here are some suggestions for improving the ocular health of your home or office:

• Ensure that your office or reading space is adequately illuminated with the appropriate illumination. There should not be excessively glaring or harsh lighting, as this can cause eye strain. If possible, relocate near a window in order to take advantage of natural light.

• To reduce reflection on your screen, you can either adjust the monitor's viewing angle or purchase an anti-glare screen protector. Position your computer and other electronic devices away from direct light.

• Adjust the luminance, contrast, and font size of the monitor for the optimal viewing experience. Reduce neck and eye strain by positioning the screen at eye level, arm's length away, and at a downward angle.

Take frequent pauses from extended screen time to rest your eyes and blink frequently. Every 20 minutes for 20 seconds, remove your eyes from the screen and focus on an object at least 20 feet distant. Blink frequently to keep your eyes lubricated and prevent them from drying out.

• Maintain proper ergonomics to reduce the strain on your eyes and body. Ensure that your feet are flat on the floor or reclining on a footrest, and that the heights of your chair and desk are appropriate. Maintain a healthy posture by using a chair designed for that purpose.

• Minimize Visual Distractions: Cover or remove anything that may cause you to lose concentration or fatigue your eyes. If your desk is neat and organized, it will be simpler to concentrate and easier on the eyes.

• Maintain hydration throughout the day by consuming copious amounts of water. Hydration is essential for preventing dehydrated eyes and maintaining healthy vision.

• Eye-Healthy Activities During Breaks: During breaks, it's a good idea to do something that won't fatigue your eyes. Try closing your eyes or performing minor eye relaxation exercises to refresh and refocus your vision.

- Clean, well-ventilated air is essential for optimal health, so maintain a clean environment. Utilize an air purifier if pollen or allergens are causing you to experience eye irritation.

- Finally, it's essential to schedule routine visits to the optometrist or ophthalmologist to have your eyes examined, have any issues corrected, and receive individualized recommendations for maintaining healthy vision.

The health of your eyes can be enhanced by making the surrounding environment more aesthetically pleasing.

CHAPTER THREE
Vision Exercises

Eye exercises consist of conducting specific motions and procedures to improve eye health and reduce eye strain. Following are some of the most important guidelines to adhere to when performing eye exercises:

• Eye exercises are more effective if they are preceded by a brief warm-up. Warm your hands by massaging them together, then rest them for a few minutes on your closed eyes. This improves blood circulation to the eyes and relaxes the eye muscles.

- Breathing and Relaxation Techniques: Before and after your eye exercises, take some time to breathe thoroughly and relax your muscles. Physical and mental relaxation can enhance the effectiveness of exercise and the general health.

- Sit comfortably in an erect position while performing eye exercises. Correct posture indirectly benefits the eyes by reducing pressure on the neck, shoulders, and back.

- Many eye exercises involve shifting your attention from one object to another that is either closer or farther away. The result is enhanced mobility and coordination of the eye muscles. First, gaze at something nearby for a few seconds, followed by something distant for a few seconds. This should be repeated numerous times.

• Eye exercises, such as eye rolls, are frequently performed due to their positive effects on eye health and function. Eye movements should include up and down, side to side, and all around. Instead of straining your eyes, perform these eye rolls slowly and evenly.

It has been demonstrated that incorporating palming, a method of tension relief, into eye exercises improves visual acuity. Rub your palms together to warm them, and then place them gently on your closed eyes. Allow the darkness and heat to sweep over you. This has the potential to alleviate eye strain and discomfort.

• Eye strain can be relieved by performing a few simple blinking exercises. To prevent your eyes from drying out, you should blink swiftly for several seconds. It may be beneficial to remind yourself to blink frequently if you find yourself gazing at a screen for extended periods.

• Concentrating on objects at varying distances is an essential element of near-to-far exercises. Examine something close up, such as your finger or a pen, and then something far away, such as a wall or a tree. Repetition of the technique improves the adjustment of the focal point.

• Regularity and Consistency In order to reap the full benefits of eye exercises, they must be performed on a consistent and regular basis. Invest at least a few minutes per day, and preferable more, in eye exercises.

• While performing eye exercises, it is essential to pay attention to your body and the signals your eyes provide. You should either slow down or cease exercising if you are experiencing pain. Consult a doctor if you have any doubts or concerns about your eyesight.

Remember that although eye exercises can benefit many individuals, they cannot replace medical care. If you have been experiencing persistent or severe vision problems, an optometrist or ophthalmologist can examine your eyes thoroughly and prescribe treatment.

Tension-And-Strress-Relieving Exercises

Eye exercises that emphasize relaxation and tension relief are an excellent way to give your eyes a break from the day's strain. Here are enumerated some common practices.

Palming is a common technique for eye relaxation. Rub your palms together to relax and warm up. To warm your eyes, make a cup with your hands and position it over your closed eyes. Take some deep breaths and close your eyes while visualizing a dark, comfortable place. Maintain this position for a few minutes to rest your eyes.

• An eye massage can reduce tension and increase blood flow to the eye area. Lightly circularly massage the skin surrounding your closed eyelids with your fingertips. Start at the center of the eye and proceed outward. Continue massaging the brow bone, temples, and eyelids for a few minutes.

• Regular blinking exercises can alleviate eye discomfort and dryness. Relax in a chair and rapidly blink your eyes for a few seconds. Then, close your eyes and don't open them for a few seconds. Repeat this process multiple times, paying particular attention to making each blink seamless and complete.

• Eye-rolling exercises can aid in increasing eye flexibility and relieving tension in the eye muscles. Relax by sitting with your eyes open and gently rolling them in a circle, first clockwise, then counterclockwise. Repeat this a number of times, avoiding eye strain by maintaining a steady, even cadence.

• Focusing from close to far is a good method to train your eyes to be more adaptable and to focus on objects at varying distances more quickly and easily.

Choose anything visible and focus on it for a while. Then, focus your gaze on the distant horizon for a while. Multiple times, use local and distant objects in this manner.

• Tracing a figure-eight shape with your gaze improves eye coordination and relaxation. Imagine an enormous number eight ten to fifteen feet in front of you. Eyes should follow the figure eight's path steadily and comfortably. Repeat this exercise several times.

• Deep breathing exercises can benefit not only the lungs, but also the pupils, which can become more relaxed. Relax and take several deep breaths while quietly seated. Fill your lungs completely with oxygen by inhaling deeply through your nose and exhaling slowly through your mouth. Focus on your breathing, and relax with each out inhalation.

Always be aware of your body and avoid placing unnecessary strain on your eyes during these activities. Immediately cease the workout and consult an eye doctor if you experience pain or discomfort.

These eye exercises can help alleviate eye strain and tension with regular practice.

CHAPTER FOUR
Coordination And Tracking Of The Eyes

The objective of visual tracking and coordination drills is to train the eyes to coordinate more effectively and monitor moving targets. These exercises have the potential to increase eye-hand coordination, strengthen eye muscles, and make concentration simpler. You can attempt the following exercises:

• To practice finger tracking, extend your arm and watch your extended index finger. Concentrate on your finger as you move it steadily in a circle, up and down and all around.

Observe your finger to ensure that your movements are in sync. As you become accustomed to the motion, speed it up and increase your range of motion.

• To practice tracking a small ball or other object, such as a pen, hold it at arm's length in front of you. Instead of moving your head, move the ball up and down, to the left and right, diagonally, and in circles.

Track the movement of the ball with your gaze without turning your head. Try to maintain a steady, unwavering focus on the objective.

• Tracking the Letters or Words: Choose a Prolonged Sentence or Word from a Book or Periodical. Position your finger beneath the word, and then move it slowly along the text while following its movement with your gaze. Attempt to effortlessly follow the path of your finger with your gaze. This activity is advantageous to both reading ability and eye-hand coordination.

• Develop hand-eye coordination by manipulating a pencil or a ball with one hand. Reach out in front of you and focus on the object you are observing.

The object is flung from one hand to the other while the observer visually tracks its movement. The object should be caught and released with precision and without jerkiness.

• Participate in visual tracking games in which on-screen or real-world characters or objects must be followed. This can be used, for example, to track the flight of a bird or the path of a bouncing object in a video game. This method of practicing eye-hand coordination can be both entertaining and beneficial.

It is essential to start slowly and gradually progress to more difficult versions of the exercises. Avoid subjecting your eyes or body to unnecessary tension. If you have preexisting eye diseases or concerns, you should consult your eye doctor prior to undertaking these exercises. Visual monitoring and coordination are abilities that can be developed with practice.

Computer Vision Syndrome Exercises

Computer Vision Syndrome (CVS) exercises are designed to alleviate eye strain induced by prolonged computer use. Try these exercises to alleviate the discomfort caused by CVS:

• Blinking Exercises: Dry, irritated eyes are a common side effect of prolonged computer screen viewing. Every few minutes, make sure to blink vigorously for a few seconds to prevent your eyes from drying out. The 20-20-20 rule recommends taking 20-second breaks every 20 minutes to look at an object at least 20 feet distant and blink normally.

• Using the palming technique, relax your eyes and relieve tension. After rubbing your hands together, cover your closed eyes with heated palms.

Place your hands over your eyes and cup them gently to block out the light. Relax by taking several deep breaths and visualizing a dark, silent room. Try palming for a few minutes if you need to rest your eyes during pauses.

• Relax your eyes and increase the range of motion of your eye muscles with these eye exercises. Examine a nearby object for a few seconds, then a distant object for the same period of time. This should be repeated numerous times. Additionally, you can relax and extend your eye muscles by rolling your eyes both clockwise and counterclockwise.

• Muscle tension in the neck and shoulders may contribute to eye fatigue. Simple exercises for the neck and shoulders can help you decompress, increase blood flow, and concentrate. Try some gentle neck adjustments to relax, such as rolling your shoulders or tilting your head to the side.

• Correcting Your Posture: Correcting your posture while using a computer can alleviate eye strain. Maintain your back against the chair and your feet on the ground. You should maintain your monitor at a comfortable distance and at eye level to avoid neck and eye strain.

• If working on a computer causes you to experience eye strain, consider adjusting the contrast and brightness settings. Choose a luminosity level that complements the ambiance, somewhere in the middle of the two extremes. Ensure that text is legible and that the screen resolution is sufficient.

• For optimal visibility, you should avoid harsh or very glaring lighting. To reduce reflections, position your monitor away from windows and other sources of direct light. By drawing the blinds or closing the draperies, you can shield your screen from the sun's glare.

Remember to take breaks when working on a computer for extended durations. Utilize the downtime to perform eye exercises, such as blinking or gazing at distant objects, to rest your eyes. Additionally, you may use an ergonomic chair and set up your workstation so that you do not have to strain your eyes, neck, or shoulders while working.

These exercises may be beneficial, but they cannot replace regular eye exams, the 20-20-20 rule, and a well-balanced diet and lifestyle if you wish to maintain your eyes' health over the long term. If your CVS symptoms are severe or persistent, consult an eye care specialist for personalized advice and treatment options.

CHAPTER FIVE
Methods For Blinking And Eye-Moisturizer Application

Preventing dryness and maintaining adequate lubrication of the eyes requires regular blinking and other methods of eye hydration. Here are a few ways to prevent your eyes from becoming dry:

• Individuals blink less frequently when engaged in activities requiring close visual attention, such as computer use. Increase the frequency of your blinks on purpose. When you blink, your tears are distributed over a larger surface area, preventing your eyes from drying out.

• When blinking, take care to give your eyes a decent, lengthy break. To qualify as a thorough blink, the eyes must be completely closed and then reopened. This motion enhances the lubrication of the eye by equitably dispersing tears across its surface.

• If your eyes continue to feel dry, use artificial tears or lubricating eye drops. The added hydration from the eye drops can temporarily alleviate discomfort in the eyes. Consult an ophthalmologist or purchase eye solutions designed for dry eyes if you experience symptoms of dry eyes.

• Warm compresses placed over closed eyelids can stimulate the production of tears and increase the flow of natural lubrication.

• A clean cloth should be soaked in warm (not boiling) water before being wrung out. Place the tepid compress on your closed eyelids and allow it to remain there for several minutes. Repeat as necessary if the dryness continues.

• Insufficiently humidified indoor air contributes to dried eyes. At home or in the office, a humidifier will add moisture to the air. This can prevent your eyes from becoming overly dry by reducing the amount of tears that evaporate.

• Smoke and pollen can irritate the eyes and make them appear even drier. It is essential to protect your eyes from smoke, airflow, and air conditioning as much as possible. When walking outside, protect your eyes from the sun and elements by wearing sunglasses or goggles.

• Adequate hydration is essential for overall eye health. Be sure to consume plenty of water throughout the day in order to reduce the likelihood of experiencing dry eyes.

Always consult an eye doctor for a thorough evaluation and treatment if you experience persistent or severe dryness, irritation, or vision changes. On the basis of your condition and their assessment of your requirements, they can provide recommendations that are unique to you.

Exercises Offer Dry Eye Relief

Eye exercises may be beneficial for dry eyes because they increase tear production, stimulate tissues that provide lubrication, and reduce eye strain. The following eye exercises are beneficial for dry-eye sufferers:

• Frequent blinking is the best method to ensure that tears are evenly distributed across the surface of the eyes. Try blinking consciously for a few seconds every 10 to 20 minutes if you have difficulty maintaining focus while performing tasks like reading or typing. This aids in maintaining a healthy tear film by restoring its moisture.

• Eye-rotation exercises can alleviate dry eye symptoms by increasing tear production. While seated, roll your eyes steadily both clockwise and counterclockwise. Repeat numerous times while maintaining even and constant movement. Try to relax your eye muscles and activate your tear ducts.

- Palming is a proven stress-relieving activity that increases tear production and reduces eye fatigue. After rubbing your hands together, cover your closed eyes with heated palms.

Create a quiet, dark environment by cupping your palms. Maintain this position while you breathe profoundly and relax for a few minutes. Palming may alleviate dryness by stimulating the production of healthful tear film.

• By alternating between near and far objects, dry eye symptoms can be alleviated and tear production can be increased. Choose a nearby object and fixate on it for a few seconds. Then, gaze far away and do the same. Repeat this multiple times to improve your eyes' ability to focus and stimulate tear production.

• Massaging the eyelids and the area surrounding the eyes stimulates the tissues responsible for producing tears. Apply a light circular pressure to your closed eyelids with your fingertips. First, concentrate on the area around the inner corner of the eye.

• Use gentle pressure, but avoid squeezing. Try this massage for a few minutes of alleviation from dryness and to stimulate tear production.

• Applying a tepid compress to the eyes may alleviate dryness and stimulate tear production. A clean cloth should be soaked in warm (not boiling) water before being wrung out. Place the tepid compress on your closed eyelids and allow it to remain there for several minutes. The oil glands are loosened by the heat, and tear production is stimulated.

• Be careful not to strain your eyes when performing these tasks. Regularly caring for your eyes entails actions such as consuming enough water, resting your eyes while performing tasks that are taxing on them, and avoiding dryness-inducing environments.

If your dry eye symptoms persist or worsen over time, you should visit an eye doctor for a thorough diagnosis and treatment plan.

CHAPTER SIX
Neck And Shoulder Strengthening Exercises

If you experience tightness or discomfort in your upper back, shoulders, or neck, try performing some stretches. These stretches may be beneficial for people who spend a lot of time sitting at a desk or engaging in activities that involve repetitive motions. Try these various forms of stretches:

- Neck rolls necessitate a comfortable position with a straight spine. Slowly rotate your head to the right, bringing your right ear to your right shoulder and your chin to your torso. As you turn your head back, bring your left ear to your left shoulder by bringing your head around. Change direction after a number of revolutions in one direction.

• To perform neck tilts, situate your head in a neutral, front-facing position. Put the right ear near to the right shoulder and incline the head to the right.

• Hold this position for 15 to 30 seconds before returning to the center. To extend the opposite side, turn the head to the left and bring the ear to the shoulder. This should be repeated multiple times on both sides.

• Rotate your shoulders while seated or standing with your arms at your sides. Slowly rotating your shoulders up and back and down and forward will relax your upper back.

• Turn in one direction for a time before reversing direction. Shoulder shrugs consist of drawing the shoulders toward the ears and then lowering them.

• Extend the right arm across the torso until it is parallel to the ground. This is a stretch for the shoulders. You can feel a stretch in the rear of your right shoulder if you bring your right arm toward you with your left hand. Stretch your right arm over your chest for 15 to 30 seconds, then move to your left arm and repeat.

• Sit or stand erect with your back straight in order to perform this stretch for the upper trapezius. Reach your right arm over your head and position your right hand on the left side of your skull to gently tilt your head to the right.

• The left side of your neck and shoulder should feel stretched.

Stretch for 15 to 30 seconds on each side before rotating.

• Levator Scapulae Stretch: While seated or standing, maintain an erect posture. Tilt your head to the left so that your left ear points toward your left shoulder. You can enhance the stretch along the right side of your neck by gently pressing down with your left hand on the side of your head. Maintain this position for 15 to 30 seconds, then alternate sides.

Always remember to stretch slowly and gently, without abrupt or forceful movements. Immediately discontinue these exercises if you experience pain or discomfort, and consult a physician.

Vision Instruction For Seniors

Eye exercises designed for the elderly can help maintain and even improve eyesight. Thanks to these activities, eye muscles will be strengthened, concentration will improve, and coordination will be refined. The following are examples of beneficial exercises for seniors:

• Practice near- and far-focus by bringing an object in and out of focus with your near hand, such as a pen. Observe it intently for a few seconds, and then shift your focus to an object in the distance for the same amount of time. Continue to shift your focus between nearby and distant objects. This exercise strengthens and makes the ocular muscles more flexible.

• The representation of the figure eight is a large horizontal figure eight in front of you. Trace the outline of the imaginary figure eight with your eyes using a steady, even motion. This activity is beneficial for the pupils' tracking and focusing abilities.

• Practicing eye-hand coordination is facilitated by holding a ball or stylus in one hand. Reach out in front of you and focus on the object you are observing.

• Observe the object as it is tossed back and forth between your palms. This activity is excellent for improving eye-hand coordination and monitoring.

• Select an image from a book or magazine to play the visual memory game. Close your eyes and visualize as much of the image as you can recall after observing it for only a few seconds.

Examine the actual object as opposed to imagining it in your mind. This mental exercise is excellent for enhancing concentration and visual memory.

• To exercise your peripheral vision, locate a comfortable seat and stare straight ahead. Focus your attention on the topic at hand while maintaining peripheral vision awareness. The exercise improves visual acuity and peripheral vision.

• By training one's eyes to move in a variety of orientations, flexibility and coordination can be improved. Maintain constant eye movement in all directions (up, down, laterally, and in circles).

Make these eye movements as naturally as feasible. This exercise can keep your eyeballs moving in multiple directions and enhance your visual agility.

Remember that you should ease into these regimens and increase the difficulty only when you are ready. Wear your glasses or contacts for the greatest possible visual experience during these activities. If you have preexisting eye conditions or concerns, the best individual to advise you on how to care for your eyes is a professional eye doctor or optician.

In addition to the benefits of eye exercises, maintaining a healthy lifestyle, including a balanced diet, staying hydrated, and engaging in regular exercise, will help ensure that your eyes remain healthy and functional as you age.

CHAPTER SEVEN
Including Eye Care Exercises In Your Routine.

Regular eye exercises are effective for maintaining and enhancing eye health. Follow these instructions to make eye exercises a regular part of your routine:

• Make a note in your calendar of when you need to perform eye exercises. To ensure that you take pauses and perform eye exercises, you could use your phone or a calendar to set reminders. This will help you develop the habit of incorporating them into your routine activities.

• Use in Conjunction with Breaks: Eye exercises can be utilized as a welcome diversion from gazing at a computer screen or engaging in other visually taxing activities.

• Perform a few minutes of eye exercises every 20 to 30 minutes. This is a welcome opportunity to take a pause from your work and rest your eyes.

• Eye exercises should be performed whenever practicable during breaks throughout the day. Consider performing eye exercises while waiting for a meeting to begin, during your commute home, or before slumber. Scene changes are an excellent time to get some exercise and rest your eyes.

• Participate in eye exercises with family or close acquaintances as a social activity. It could be a social gathering where you support one another. Schedule regular gatherings where you can all perform the exercises and discuss your progress.

• Make Minor Adjustments: Include Eye Exercises in Your Daily Routine. Try performing simple eye movements or concentration shifts, similar to when you brush your teeth.

Utilize your stoplight time to practice eye relaxation techniques. You can incorporate eye exercises into your routine more readily if you incorporate them into already established practices.

• Keep Your Posture in Mind: When performing eye exercises, it is essential to keep your posture in mind. Maintain a straight alignment between your cranium and spine. When you maintain proper posture, your blood circulates more efficiently and your eye muscles function at their peak.

• Incorporate eye exercises with other stress-reduction techniques, such as deep breathing or meditation. This has the additional benefit of calming your entire mind and body, not just your pupils.

• Maintain Consistency If you want results from your eye exercises, you must perform them consistently. Commit to performing eye exercises frequently, ideally every day. Maintaining a regular schedule will result in gradual improvements to your eyesight.

Consider that your particular needs and time constraints will necessitate modifying these suggestions. As your eye muscles become stronger and your range of motion increases, you can progress to more challenging tasks. If you have any preexisting eye conditions or concerns, we can help.

Conquering Obstacles And Maintaining Motivation

It may be necessary to overcome obstacles and maintain motivation in order to obtain the benefits of eye exercises. Here are some techniques to help you persevere during difficult times:

• Goal-Setting It is essential to commence eye exercises with a set of objectives in mind. You must divide your objectives into more manageable pieces. Recognizing and rewarding your efforts along the way may maintain your enthusiasm and dedication.

• Keep track of your exercises and note any changes that occur as a result of your efforts. Keeping track of your workout progress is as simple as using a calendar or a mobile app. Keeping a visual record of your accomplishments is a fantastic way to stay motivated and proud of your accomplishments.

• Develop your eye exercise routine with a friend, relative, or colleague who shares your interest. Maintain each other's integrity and motivation to stick to a routine.

Share your struggles and victories with one another to encourage and motivate one another.

• Make it Fun: Think of creative ways to make eye exercises enjoyable. Listen to soothing music, practice in an environment where you feel comfortable, or incorporate things you appreciate, such as imagining happy scenes or employing vibrant visual aids. If workouts are pleasant, it will be easier to maintain motivation.

• Keep your routines interesting by varying your eye exercises on occasion. This helps exercise multiple eye muscles and reduces the likelihood of monotony. Experiment with various forms of exercise to discover the ones that suit you best and to keep your routine interesting.

• Instead of viewing eye exercises as additional labor, make them a regular part of your break schedule. Develop the habit of taking frequent breaks to rest your eyes and preserve their health. Frequent pauses are associated with decreased instances of eye strain and increased productivity.

• Seek Assistance and Resources: Seek assistance and resources that can serve as inspiration and guidance. Participate in online forums or communities with individuals who value eye health. Consult an eye doctor who can tailor their recommendations to your specific requirements and closely monitor your progress.

• Consider the benefits of conducting frequent eye exercises. Consider the advantages they will provide for your eyes, such as the ability to rest your eyes more easily, to concentrate better, and to maintain clear vision. Consider how far your efforts will reach in the future.

• Don't be so harsh on yourself if you miss a day or struggle to maintain consistency. Obstacles are inevitable on any voyage. Always remember that you are making progress, however small. Be kind to yourself and rededicate yourself to your training without punishing yourself for errors.

If you apply these strategies and remain committed to your objective, you can maintain and improve your eye health through regular eye exercises.

CHAPTER EIGHT
Promoting Eye Health Through Diet And Exercise

However, adopting a healthier lifestyle may have a greater impact on your acuity. Following are some suggestions:

• Consume a balanced diet that includes eye-healthy items in order to maintain optimal vision. Consume plenty of vitamin A, vitamin C, vitamin E, and omega-3 fatty acid-rich produce. Some examples include greens, vegetables, oranges, berries, nuts, seeds, and fish. A balanced diet can provide the necessary nutrients for maintaining healthy eyes.

• Consume copious amounts of water throughout the day to maintain hydration. Maintaining tear production and preventing dehydrated eyes can be accomplished by consuming sufficient water.

• Professionals in the field of optometry advise regular comprehensive eye exams. When you receive regular eye exams, any vision problems or changes can be detected and treated more effectively.

• The 20-20-20 rule is an effective guideline for reducing eye strain caused by screen use. Every 20 minutes, you should take a 20-second break to stare at something at least 20 feet distant. Aspects of screen ergonomics include seated at the correct distance from the computer and utilizing the proper lighting.

• Wearing sunglasses that block 100 percent of UV radiation is the most effective method to protect your eyes from the sun's damaging rays when you're outdoors. Cataracts and other eye diseases are less likely to form, and the delicate tissues of the eye are protected.

• Restful Sleep: Make sleep a consistent part of your regimen. You can reduce eye strain and improve the overall health of your eyes by getting sufficient rest.

• If you are currently a smoker, kindly consider quitting. Cigarette smoking has been linked to several eye diseases and disorders, including macular degeneration and cataracts. If you care about your eyesight, you must cease smoking.

• Establish safeguards to protect your eyes from injury. Protective eyewear is required for sports, do-it-yourself projects, and working with potentially hazardous materials. Eye injuries caused by trauma can have enduring effects on eyesight.

• Work with your physician to determine the most effective method to manage chronic health conditions such as diabetes and hypertension. Managing these conditions can prevent complications, including eye injury.

• Avoiding tension is essential for your eyes and overall health. Engage in activities that help you decompress and relax, such as exercise, meditation, deep breathing, or your favorite pastime.

You can supplement the benefits of eye exercises and enhance your overall eye health by incorporating these changes into your daily routine. Remember that the secret to excellent eye health is a combination of a healthy lifestyle and routine professional care.

The Conclusion

Regular eye exercises are necessary for maintaining and improving visual acuity. They can aid in the reduction of eye fatigue, the development of robust eye muscles, the improvement of concentration, coordination, and adaptability, as well as the enhancement of overall visual health.

Make eye exercises a part of your daily regimen to support your eyes and reduce your risk of common eye diseases.

It is essential to create an eye-friendly environment, prepare for exercises, and adhere to the fundamentals of eye exercises for effective practice. Exercises for relaxation, visual tracking, and coordination, as well as computer vision syndrome, assist with common eye problems.

In addition to targeted eye exercises, a more comprehensive approach to eye health is required. A healthy lifestyle includes eating well, drinking enough water, having regular eye exams, protecting your eyes from the sun, using electronic devices properly, treating chronic illnesses, and reducing stress.

If you make these modifications to your daily routine, you can enhance your overall eye health and get the most out of your eye exercises.

Remember that the keys to successfully incorporating eye exercises and lifestyle changes into your daily routine are consistency, setting reasonable goals, monitoring progress, seeking assistance, and remaining motivated. You can have clear vision and healthy eyes as long as you give your eyes the care they deserve as part of your regular self-care routine.

THE END

48660CB00001B/491